Proactive Stress Management
Optimizing Your Position in the River of Life

Dave Chong, PhD

DEDICATION

To Irving Zola (1935-1994), whose river story inspired this book.

.

ABOUT THE AUTHOR

Dave is a faculty member in health sciences, teaching courses in Stress Management, Wellness, Health Assessments, Anatomy & Physiology, Medical Terminology, and Research Methods. He holds a Ph.D. in Health Promotion & Education, a Master's in Exercise & Wellness, and certifications from the American College of Sports Medicine, the Wilderness Medicine Institute, and the National Registry of Emergency Medical Technicians.

TABLE OF CONTENTS

Introduction

It's easy to read scientific studies about stress and well-being. It's *not* easy to see stress ravaging the lives of your students, clients, friends, and family members, along with personally experiencing those same outcomes in your own life.

In my role as a wellness educator, stress has consistently been the single most substantial issue affecting the lives of the people with whom I work, and it affects them in *every* wellness dimension (i.e., physically, intellectually, emotionally, socially, spiritually, occupationally, and environmentally). In fact, when people seek professional advice about changing their physical health behaviors (e.g., actions relating to alcohol, food, tobacco, physical inactivity, etc.), they often find that *non*-physical factors like stress are actually the driving force behind their physical behaviors. As a result, optimal stress management has both direct and indirect effects on improving a person's quality of life.

Beginning with the first page in Chapter 1, you'll also soon discover that my interest in this topic isn't simply academic. Instead, the adverse stress outcomes I experienced over 20 years ago sparked a journey that has since transformed not only my own life, but also the lives of others. It's therefore a path I'm now grateful to have traveled, and I hope it makes your own voyage a much smoother one.

Aloha, Dave.

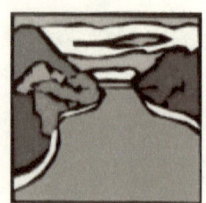

CHAPTER 1
A TRUE STORY

During my junior year of college, I almost dropped out of school because of some struggles I was having with the required coursework. My thought process at the time involved many different elements and was therefore quite complicated, and although I knew I was feeling "stressed out" about the whole thing, I didn't truly realize how much the stress was affecting me until I woke up one morning and found that my jaw was locked almost completely shut (I could only open it about a half inch).

I soon learned from my doctor that as I slept every night, my stress was manifesting itself in the form of "bruxism" (i.e., grinding of the teeth), which caused the two small discs between my jawbone and skull to dislodge, thereby locking my jaw.

For the ensuing treatment program, I was required to wear a custom-made mouth splint constantly (24/7). I was also given a bottle of liquid topical medicine (a muscle relaxer), and I had to spray the liquid onto my face several times per day and then massage the muscles surrounding my jaw. In the meantime, of course, my nutrition habits changed dramatically, because I could barely open my mouth and the act of chewing was out of the question (ultimately, I drank all of my food through straws).

Fortunately, my jaw suddenly unlocked a few weeks later, and it was the most spectacular feeling I'd ever had. Seriously, although the relief was only temporary at the time, I can't even begin to tell you how wonderful it felt to be able to open my mouth again after having it stuck closed for so long. My jaw also then gradually began to unlock at more frequent intervals and for longer durations, until it finally got to the point where it was almost back to normal (although I haven't been able to chew gum or eat any "Dagwood"-style sandwiches since).

Looking back, I certainly don't ever want to go through that experience again, and it was such a startling wake-up call that I've also been working ever since to help other people avoid the same fate. In fact, after I graduated from college (thanks to some great tutors and classmates), I went on to study stress management in graduate school, using it as the underlying topic for my thesis and dissertation. Along the way, I learned a number of things about stress that I wished I'd known a *long* time before, and it has been wonderful privilege to subsequently share those things as a wellness educator and as an instructor for undergraduate stress management courses.

Overall, the single most important insight I've gained from this journey has been realizing the difference between *proactive* stress management and *reactive* stress management, which is such a vital distinction that I'm writing this book to help other people learn all about it. More specifically, I hope the proactive principle becomes as helpful to you as it has been to me, and that you never have to spend a month drinking your food through straws in order to realize the importance of optimal stress management.

THREE QUICK QUESTIONS

Before you continue reading through this book, please stop for a moment and answer the following three questions, preferably by actually writing your answers down somewhere:

1. What is your personal definition of "stress?" (and please refrain from using any technical descriptions, so you won't sound like your high school science teacher who probably said something like: "Stress is the non-specific response of a biological organism to an outside stimulus"; instead, think about how you feel when you're "stressed out" and use *that* concept of stress to answer this first question).

2. What are the things that cause you stress? (i.e., what are your personal stressors, meaning the various things in life that make you feel stressed out?).

3. What are your stress coping strategies? (i.e., what are the things you do to alleviate your stress?).

In all sincerity, if you'll take a little time right now to stop and answer these questions before continuing on to read the rest of this book, you'll get a *lot* more out of what you're about to read.

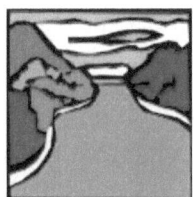

CHAPTER 2
THE RELEVANCE OF STRESS

WHAT *IS* STRESS?

The reason you were asked in the last chapter to define stress in your own words is because there are literally dozens of definitions available for "stress" today, and it's therefore important for us to establish some common ground before we continue. After all, the word "stress" can be used as both a noun and a verb, with each of those forms having several possible meanings. As a result, "stress" can represent very different things to different people (with all of those definitions being equally valid), which is why *perception* is one of the most important principles in stress education and why we'll be talking more about it in a minute.

That being said, please compare your personal definition of stress with the two interpretations shown below, both of which are very helpful for sharing stress management principles with different people from a variety of diverse backgrounds:

- The first definition is from the Merriam-Webster dictionary, in which stress is described as a form of "bodily or mental tension resulting from factors that tend to alter an existent equilibrium."

- The second definition comes from a pair of American professors (Ray & Seaward), who define stress as "a state of anxiety produced when perceived demands from events and responsibilities exceed one's perceived coping abilities, resulting in a series of physiological responses that may result in dysfunction and disease."

Okay, that second one is admittedly a mouthful, but – overall –

what do you think? Did either of those statements sound anything like your own definition? Personally, the reason I like those two descriptions is because they collectively address the six most essential elements of the human stress experience: stimuli, perceptions, coping, tension/anxiety, homeostasis, and stress outcomes. Let's review each of these major factors.

STIMULI

The formal term in stress management for a stimulus is a "stressor," which refers to any of the numerous occurrences to which our bodies are continuously exposed. Indeed, there are literally *millions* of potential stressors, because almost everything in life is a stimulus of some sort, and not necessarily in a bad way. In fact, if you stop and think about it, a total absence of stimuli is only possible if you're dead, and all humans actually need stimulation in order to feel optimally alive and energized. Therefore, scientists often classify stress and stressors as belonging to either of two main categories: "eustress" (i.e., "good stress," such as pay raises, job promotions, graduations, etc.) or "distress" (i.e., "bad" stress, such as bills you can't afford to pay, traffic jams when you're late, diagnoses of terminal diseases, and so on).

However, all stressors aren't either just good *or* bad, because a lot of things in life have the potential to be good *and* bad, depending on the intensity and timing of the stimulus. To illustrate that concept, take a look at Figure 2.1, where a stimulus (stressor) is plotted on the horizontal axis, in comparison to a vertical plot for well-being (which is the simultaneous status of your physical, intellectual, emotional, social, spiritual, occupational, and environmental health).

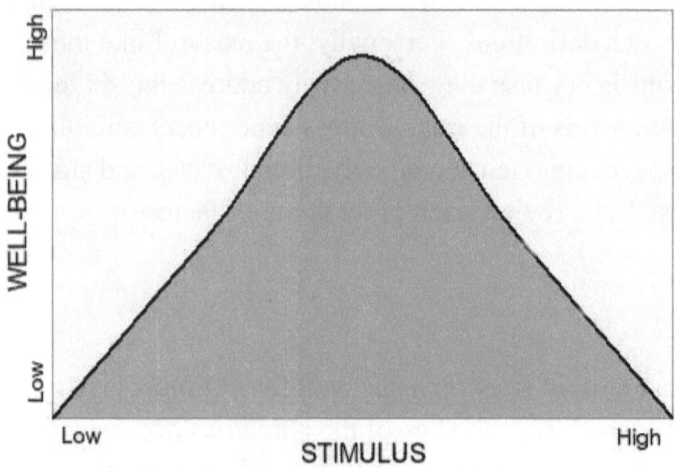

Figure 2.1 – Stimulus (Stressor) Curve

While you're looking at the Stimulus Curve, mentally replace the word "Stimulus" on the horizontal axis with the name of a specific stimulus from your own life. For example, various stimuli from throughout the wellness spectrum include: work, food, sleep, news, affection, money, sunlight, etc. Then, using your selected stimulus to compare the Stimulus Curve to the life experiences you've already had, you'll probably see the meaning of the graph pretty quickly, because it shows that when you have the right amounts of life's different stimuli (i.e., not too much or too little, depending on your individual needs and preferences), your personal well-being and quality of life are genuinely optimized, in the same way that Goldilocks was finally able to sleep soundly once she found a bed that was "just right."

On the other hand, though, if you have too much or too little of life's various stimuli, your well-being and quality of life decrease substantially, even for the subtle things you don't always think about (e.g., ambient temperature changes, personal hydration status, etc.). And you already know that's true if you've ever had too much or too little food…too much or too little sleep…too much or too little work…etc. All of which goes to show that stimuli always have to be present in order for your stress response to be activated, and if they occur in excessive or insufficient amounts, you may experience considerable distress.

PERCEPTION & COPING

As mentioned in the preceding section, the "right" amount of a stimulus for you won't necessarily be the right amount of that same stimulus for someone else, and vice versa. After all, human beings have a wide variety of needs and desires for food, sleep, work, money, and so on. Plus, major life events such as pregnancy, marriage, divorce, graduation, and job termination can also be interpreted very differently, depending on whether or not you wanted any of those things to happen in the first place (either entirely, or just in the way that they did). In other words, you're simply not going to feel distressed in situations which don't matter or apply to you.

Speaking of which, take a look back at the 2nd question you were asked in the first chapter. Specifically, what is it about your personal stressors that *does* matter and apply to you? And *why?* (your answers here will offer a glimpse into some of your deepest personal values, as you'll soon see).

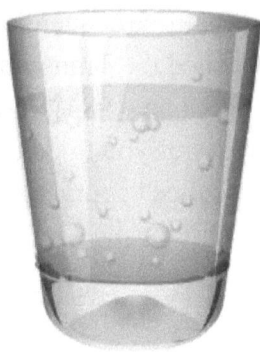

Figure 2.2 – Perception

Another factor also affecting our personal reactions to stimuli is our perceived ability to *cope* with those stimuli, because people who sense an abundance of available coping methods tend to feel much less stressed than folks whose options seem rather limited (with this situation often being described in terms of each person's "comfort zones"). In fact, if you consider each individual's unique set of coping options as being a "toolbox" of stress coping strategies, it's pretty obvious that the people who have more tools (and know how to use them) clearly have more alternatives than the folks with fewer tools.

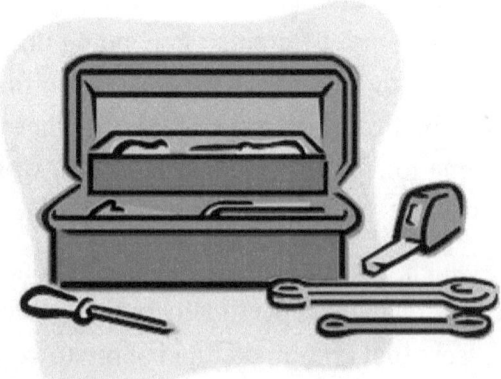

Figure 2.3 – Stress Coping Toolbox

In the academic community, these sequential stages of perception are described in a theory called the Transactional Model of Stress & Coping (Lazarus and Folkman, 1984). To put it simply, every stimulus you encounter requires you to go through at least one of two perceptual processes (called "appraisals"), each of which may occur consciously or subconsciously:

- <u>Primary Appraisal</u> – does this situation *matter and apply* to me?

- <u>Secondary Appraisal</u> – if this situation does matter and apply to me, what *options* do I have for responding to it?

During the first appraisal, if a stimulus doesn't matter or apply to you then you're certainly not going to identify it as a stressful one, and you therefore won't be concerned about your available coping options or your potential for feeling distress. Conversely, if the stimulus does matter and apply to you, then you'll progress into the secondary appraisal, in which you'll determine how well-equipped you are for coping with that stressor. Let's use the random topic of sharks for a few practical examples:

- Example #1 – You're deathly afraid of sharks. However, you live in Nebraska and have never even been to an aquarium (much less an ocean), so your stress process won't go any further than the primary appraisal, because sharks don't inhabit corn fields and their presence doesn't *apply* to you.

- Example #2 – You're an ocean swimmer who lives in Hawaii, but you love sharks and think they're cute. As a result, your stress process will also stop at the primary appraisal, because the stimulus doesn't *matter* to you, even though it applies to you.

- Example #3 – You're another ocean swimmer who lives in Hawaii, but you're terrified of sharks, which means you'll determine in your primary appraisal that sharks do matter and apply to you. You'll therefore also conduct a secondary appraisal in order to establish the number of *options* you have for swimming safely, and your ultimate distress level will be "inversely proportional" to the number of options you perceive. In other words, the more tools you have in your stress coping toolbox, the lower your level of distress will be.

This integral role of perception in stress is actually one of the key reasons why it's possible for you to receive contradictory results from different stress "surveys" (i.e., stress questionnaires in magazines, research studies, etc.), because they all ask about stress in unique ways, with some surveys focusing primarily on the presence or absence of certain stimuli, and others focusing instead on your perceptions of those stimuli. Also, some surveys focus exclusively on either short-term ("acute") or long-term ("chronic") stress, while others focus only on coping strategies.

For instance, the *The Holmes-Rahe Life Stress Inventory* and the *Personal Stress Inventory* are two very different stress surveys, and they're mentioned here simply to emphasize that there really isn't any such thing as the one and only "correct" stress questionnaire. Instead, because all stress surveys focus on different stress factors, it's entirely possible for you to answer several different surveys and receive conflicting "scores" for all of them. That's a very important point to make here, because health professionals routinely hear clients say things like, "Oh no! I took a stress survey in a magazine, and it told me that I'm totally stressed out!"

Listen, if you need a survey to tell you that you're stressed out, then you're really not as stressed as you think you are. Plus, it's very challenging for scientists to create surveys which can accurately "measure" psychological attributes (e.g., stress, courage, happiness, etc.), especially when the traits they're trying to measure involve perceptions. Please keep these things in mind the next time you fill out a stress survey, because now you know that your personal stress response is dependent on multiple perceptual factors.

You might also like to know that perception is one of the things most commonly addressed by successful stress management programs. That's because feelings of distress are dramatically reduced when you realize that certain stimuli don't actually matter as much as you previously thought they did, and/or when you add more stress coping strategies to your toolbox.

TENSION / ANXIETY

If a stressor occurs which you perceive to be relevant, *and* if you feel you don't have a well-stocked toolbox of stress coping strategies, you'll enter a phase of uneasiness which results from being displaced from your comfort zone. This is particularly true if you believe the situation's demands exceed your coping abilities, thereby also introducing the additional factor of *worrying*, which results in more uneasiness, more worrying, and so on. All of this leads to tension (feeling mentally or emotionally strained) and/or anxiety (feeling worried, nervous, or uneasy), each of which can completely wreak havoc on your body.

Of course, at this point you might be thinking, "Hey, I don't know what you're talking about. I worry about stuff all the time, but otherwise I feel fine." And sure, that may be true *for now*, but be very careful about falling for the old "if-it-doesn't-hurt-it's-okay" myth. A lot of people do all sorts of things that are – in one way or another (i.e., physically, emotionally, occupationally, etc.) – unmistakably harmful to them in the long run, and yet they don't realize the presence of danger because their actions only affect them a little bit at a time. Then, five or ten years later when they "suddenly" suffer a physical or emotional breakdown due to all of the accumulated damage, they don't recognize the true origin of their demise because everything seemed to be fine for so long. That's why it's so important to introduce the topic of "homeostasis" here.

HOMEOSTASIS

Homeostasis is a Greek word that's often translated as "standing still," and it's used in the science of physiology to describe your body's relentless efforts to maintain a *constant internal condition regardless of external stimuli.* For instance, two obvious examples of human homeostasis are your body's temperature and hydration status, both of which are continuously being fine-tuned to stay within certain acceptable ranges, despite external variables such as the weather, your clothing, the amounts and types of beverages and foods you've consumed, etc. In other words, the process of homeostasis acts a lot like the thermostat in your house, working constantly to keep your internal environment the same, regardless of what's happening outside.

From the standpoint of stress management, homeostasis is a very important topic because – just as with temperature and hydration – your body also has an ideal balance between the amount of time it spends performing hard work and the amount of time it spends resting. And during each of those periods, your nervous system and your endocrine (hormone) system send signals to your body's organs (e.g., heart, lungs, stomach, kidneys, etc.), causing those organs to either work harder or rest easier in order to maintain homeostasis and optimize your well-being.

So far, so good, right? After all, it makes perfect sense that you and your organs need to work hard at certain times and take it easy at other times, so that everything stays in balance. You might not realize, however, that your body automatically switches into the hard work mode *every* time you encounter a stressor and perceive it to be relevant, because no matter what the stressor is (e.g., tax bill, computer failure, big hairy spider, etc.), your body always reacts by activating the legendary "fight-or-flight" response. And that would actually be okay if your stressors were infrequent and therefore allowed you to fully rest and recuperate between each stimulus. However, our modern "go-go-go!" lifestyles have unfortunately immersed us in a 24/7 non-stop stream of continuous stimulation, which is then amplified by our pesky human habit of constantly worrying about our stressors.

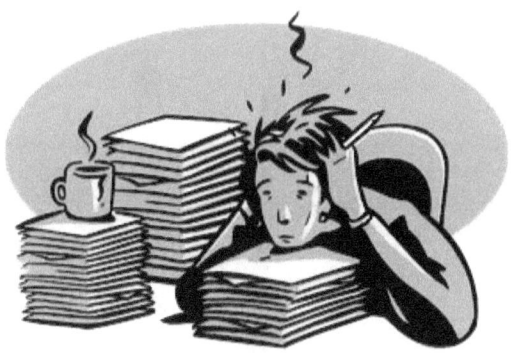

Figure 2.4 – Chronic Stressor

So instead of facing occasional, well-spaced stimuli separated by ample rest periods, we pile on the stressors from the time we wake up in the morning until the time we collapse asleep at night, which completely obliterates our body's attempts to maintain homeostasis. In addition, even when our bodies start giving us warning signs (such as fatigue, irritability, burnout, etc.) that we're transitioning from the "fight-or-flight" mode into full-on exhaustion, we blindly urge each other to keep plodding along by sharing supposedly motivational sayings like, "Suck it up!" or "Sleep when you're dead!"

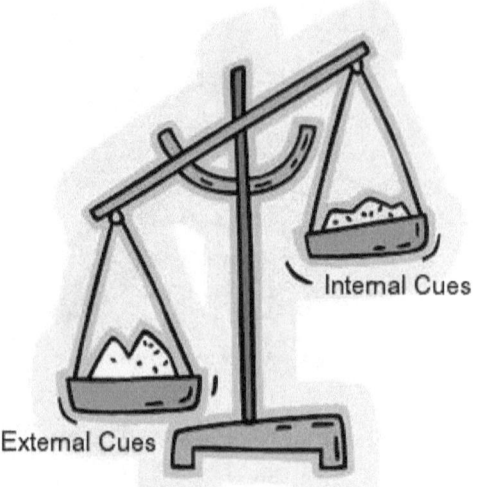

Figure 2.5 – Life Out of Balance

Unfortunately, humans eventually pay a staggering price for repeatedly prioritizing their external cues (e.g., deadlines, peer pressures, and other outside demands) over internal cues (such as the warning signs mentioned in the preceding paragraph). That's because the resulting imbalance eventually overwhelms all of the body's attempts to maintain homeostasis, resulting in a staggering number of adverse stress outcomes.

STRESS OUTCOMES

The lockjaw episode described in Chapter 1 is known in the medical world as a form of TMJ Disorder, and it's one of the many adverse health outcomes of chronic stress. Indeed, stress is also associated with cardiovascular disease, headaches, high blood pressure, insomnia, chest pain, fatigue, and a variety of other ailments, all of which clearly fit the description of "psychosomatic" (mind-body) diseases. And although it's rare to meet anyone who *wants* a decreased quality of life and an increased risk for disease and premature death, those are exactly the outcomes being experienced by the millions of chronically stressed people in this modern world. For that reason, let's explore how to optimize your approach to stress management, so you can minimize your stress and maximize your wellness.

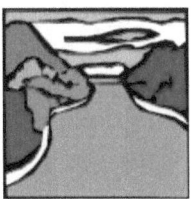

CHAPTER 3
PROACTIVE STRESS MANAGEMENT

ARE YOU UPSTREAM OR DOWNSTREAM?

One of the most famous stories shared among health educators is credited to the great medical sociologist Irving Zola (1935-1994), and it is told from the perspective of a physician frustrated by modern medical practice.

"You know," he said, "sometimes it feels like this. There I am standing by the shore of a swiftly flowing river and I hear the cry of a drowning man. So I jump into the river, put my arms around him, pull him to shore and apply artificial respiration. Just when he begins to breathe, there is another cry for help. So I jump into the river, reach him, pull him to shore, apply artificial respiration, and then just as he begins to breathe, another cry for help. So back in the river again, reaching, pulling, applying, breathing and then another yell. Again and again, without end, goes the sequence. You know, I am so busy jumping in, pulling them to shore, applying artificial respiration, that I have no time to see who the hell is upstream pushing them all in."

[McKinlay, John B. 2001. "A Case for Refocusing Upstream: The Political Economy of Illness." In *The Sociology of Health and Illness: Critical Perspectives*, 6th ed., edited by Peter Conrad, 516-29. New York: Worth Publishers.]

The moral of Zola's tale explains why *proactive* stress management is such a radically different approach than *reactive* stress management, and here's why:

- Proactive stress management: relieves distress by ***resolving the original stressor***

- <u>Reactive stress management</u>: relieves distress, but does <u>NOT</u> resolve the original stressor.

We'll look at a few examples of this difference in a moment, but before we do that, take a glance back at the 3rd question you were asked in Chapter 1. In particular, when you look at your list of stress coping strategies, which of them are *proactive* (meaning that they truly resolve at least one of the stressors listed in your answer to the 2nd question), and which of your strategies are *reactive* (meaning that they don't resolve any of your stressors, and instead only divert your attention away from those stressors)? This difference is more important than you might think.

ANGRY BIRDS

I laughed myself silly the first time I played the *Angry Birds* video game, because the game's designers have created an ingenious activity using key insights into human psychology. However, whenever I hear someone say they're going to "relieve some stress" by playing a video game, it reminds me that too many people rely almost exclusively on *reactive* stress coping strategies like that one, which ultimately inhibits them in the long run.

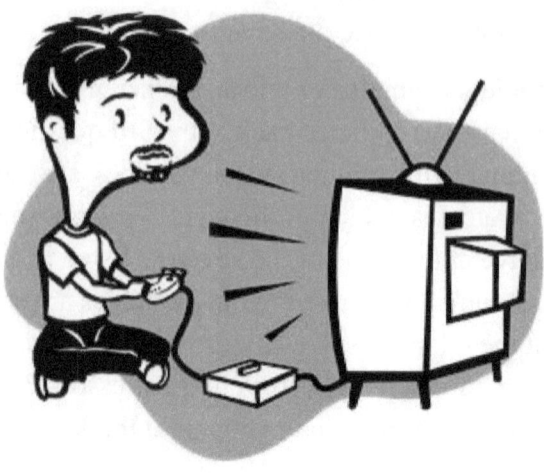

Figure 3.1 – Reactive Coping Strategy

In other words, although video games can provide wonderful entertainment (along with the development of spectacular hand-eye coordination), they're also unfortunately very effective at distracting people from higher-priority tasks. For instance, if your most significant stressor right now is an important project or assignment that's due tomorrow morning, and you choose to go play video games for two hours instead of finishing your project, you obviously haven't resolved your original stressor. In fact, you've actually made that situation *more* stressful, because you'll now have even less time available to complete the same task by the same deadline. That's a common example of reactive stress management, and here are some other classics:

Reactive Example #2: If your personal finances are currently your most relevant stressor, and you choose to deal with your distress by receiving weekly massages for $70 per hour at a nearby spa, have you resolved your original stressor? Nope! If anything, you've made it worse.

Reactive Example #3: If your relationship with a certain person (e.g., family member, coworker, neighbor, etc.) is your most relevant stressor, and you respond to that situation by drowning your distress in alcohol every night, have you resolved your original stressor? Absolutely not, because your drinking hasn't changed the underlying relationship between you and that other person, and you might even aggravate things further if the alcohol prompts you to do something regrettable.

Of course, people frequently use reactive coping strategies because those methods often provide the easiest and fastest distractions from their personal stressors. What's tragic, though, is that many stress management programs don't include *any* proactive strategies among their recommendations. It's true; far too many "stress reduction" programs are completely reactive, with strategies focused exclusively on things like physical activity and personal pampering (e.g., gym workouts, pedicures, and so on), without any use whatsoever of proactive strategies (such as conflict resolution, communication enhancement, goal-setting, etc.). Conversely, optimal stress management programs include a balance of reactive *and* proactive strategies, each of which is further described below.

SORTING YOUR STRATEGIES

Whenever working with clients and students on stress management, I always ask them the same three questions you were asked in the first chapter of this book. One reason I do that is to reinforce that the entire stress process depends on each person's own perceptions of stressors and stress coping strategies. For example, you might feel stressed by something that other folks think is insignificant, while they might feel stressed by something that you consider irrelevant. In addition, another reason I ask those questions is to see if people's stress coping methods are proactive or reactive, and here's a quick summary (in no particular order) of the strategies they most commonly include in their responses:

- Listening to music
- Playing music (as a musician)
- Golfing
- Reading
- Weight training
- Running / walking
- Spending time with family (parents / spouse / children / cousins / etc.)
- Spending time with friends
- Bicycling
- Fishing
- Skiing (water or snow)
- Surfing the Internet
- Canoeing / kayaking
- Surfing / windsurfing
- Swimming
- Hiking / climbing
- Gardening / landscaping
- Volunteering (charities / communities / etc.)
- Attending church activities (sermons / choir practice / small group meetings)
- Praying / having faith in God
- Meditating
- Breathing deeply
- Sailing / boating
- Flying (airplanes / seaplanes / gliders / remote-controlled aircraft / etc.)
- Improving houses / homes
- Restoring cars / aircraft / etc.
- Restoring furniture
- Woodworking / carving
- Hunting / shooting / archery
- Creating art
- Viewing art

- Laughing
- Singing
- Dancing
- Writing (letters / journals / creative stories / etc.)
- Playing games (video / board / recreational)
- Cooking
- Cleaning
- Knitting / sewing
- Collecting (stamps / doll houses / antiques / etc.)

Looking at the above list, how many of your own personal strategies did you see included? And, more importantly, which of those strategies would you view as being reactive, and which of them would you view as being proactive?

By this point in the book, hopefully the preceding pages have helped you to recognize that in order to label a strategy as being proactive or reactive, you first have to identify the original stressor. For instance, here are two quick examples of how a single coping method might either be proactive or reactive, depending on the circumstances:

- If your most relevant stressor is driving through rush-hour traffic, and you choose to relieve your distress by going swimming after dealing with that traffic, then that's a reactive strategy because your swim sessions aren't resolving the traffic or your ability to drive without feeling stressed. However, if your most relevant stressor is a fear of drowning, and you're taking swimming lessons so you can conquer that fear, then that's a proactive strategy because learning to swim *is* addressing your fear of drowning.

- If your relationship with your boss is currently your most relevant stressor, and you choose to relieve your distress by going fishing after you leave the office, then that would be a reactive strategy because fishing isn't changing your relationship with your boss or improving your ability to get along with that person in the future. On the other hand, if your most relevant stressor is the cost of fish at your local market, and you're going fishing so you won't have to buy any more fish at the store, then that's a proactive strategy because the price of fish won't affect you any more.

Of course, please keep in mind that some strategies (like the video games mentioned earlier) are less likely to have proactive applications, while other strategies (such as meditation and reframing) are more likely to have proactive applications.

MENTAL COPING OPTIONS

Looking back at the Transactional Model introduced in Chapter 2, you'll remember that "primary appraisals" are internal processes in which people evaluate whether or not stressors matter and apply to them. So, if you're a student who *likes* exams, or a homeowner who *likes* household repairs, or a swimmer who *likes* sharks, then those things won't matter to you from a personal distress standpoint (even when they apply to you); as a result, you won't be concerned about your available coping options or your potential for feeling distressed. That's why mental coping strategies like meditation and reframing can be so effective, because – although they may initially appear to be only reactive – they're actually also proactive because they affect the way your mind responds to stressors during primary appraisals:

- **Meditation** has existed for literally thousands of years and encompasses many different styles, including progressive relaxation, mindfulness, movement meditation, mantra repetition, and so on. In fact, there are so many forms and styles of meditation that the "best" method is simply the one that resonates most strongly with you. And regardless of which style you choose, the main benefit from all forms of meditation is an improved control over your mind, which allows you to shed regrets and worries while also responding to stressors rationally instead of emotionally. This improved self-control will allow you to calmly and appropriately assess the relevance of every stimulus you encounter, along with being able to wisely choose additional coping strategies from your stress coping toolbox, if necessary. For more information about the many different meditation techniques available, check out some of the national or international associations located in your part of the world. In the United States, for instance, the *Meditation Society of America* has a website which currently lists over 100 different meditation methods.

- **"Reframing"** refers to the mental process of looking at situations from different points of view, and it is often casually (and incompletely) described as "looking on the bright side" of things. In reality, reframing is about much more than just making a switch from pessimism to optimism. It's about – as Viktor Frankl famously described in his book about surviving Nazi concentration camps – "Man's Search for Meaning." Indeed, every situation in life (including suffering, according to Frankl and many others) offers you a meaningful occasion to learn and grow and develop, and if you use that type of mindset when responding to stressors, it will have a profoundly positive impact on you and everyone else around you. That's because once you integrate reframing into your primary appraisals, you'll soon find your life's stressors assuming an entirely different nature, in which each stimulus becomes an opportunity inspiring hope, rather than a burden bringing despair.

By the way, although reframing and meditation are both often associated with people of faith (i.e., those who believe in a divine power), they're actually applicable to everyone. A legendary example of that versatility is on vivid display in Frankl's "Man's Search for Meaning" book, in which Holocaust survivors (some of whom reframed with faith and some of whom didn't) clearly demonstrated a level of resilience that's as remarkable as any in human history.

Meanwhile, dramatic changes in your life from meditation and/or reframing may not happen overnight, but they *will* happen, and – as scientists like to say – the benefits will be directly proportional to your investment. That means the more you make use of these strategies, the better your results will be, and that's especially true for overcoming the habit of worrying (which you'll find to be a truly remarkable accomplishment in itself).

ACTIVE AND CHILDLIKE

Now, please don't be concerned if you're currently thinking, "Uh oh, I don't have any mental strategies, because my entire list of stress coping methods consists of only hands-on physical stuff." No worries!

First of all, you'll be able to add mental strategies whenever you feel ready to try them, and you'll know exactly when that time arrives because it typically happens as suddenly as the flicking of a light switch. Secondly, many of the *non*-mental strategies still utilize two especially valuable stress reduction principles: physical activity and creative personal expression.

The major benefit of **physical activity** in regards to stress management is that it exactly matches your body's "fight-or-flight" response, which you may remember from Chapter 2 as an automatic and immediate transition into a hard work mode. In other words, every time you're faced with a relevant stressor, a number of physiological changes inside your body immediately configure you to either fight for your life or run for your life (both of which are certainly very physical things). So if you respond to your stressors by being physically active, that can be an outstanding response. Please be careful to note, however, that if an *excessive* amount of physical activity or other type of hard work *is* your stressor (because of sports, job demands, etc.), then the best response in that case may be for you to be *less* active. After all, your body can only adapt to life's demands for hard work when you give it enough time to fully recuperate in between those work periods.

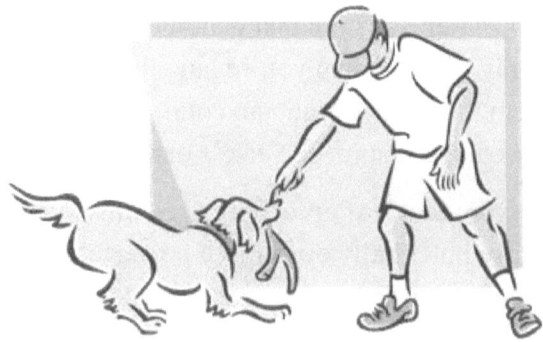

Figure 3.2 – Physical Activity

As a side note, one of the most commonly recommended physical relaxation strategies is the practice of deep breathing, and many Westerners tend to be a little skeptical about that because they don't understand its rationale. However, there are several important features of deep breathing, and they include:

- Affordability – unlike many stress reduction methods which require some sort of financial expenditure, breathing is free.

- Availability – you can breathe deeply just about anywhere, because your breath goes wherever you go.

- <u>Relaxation</u> – deep breathing stimulates your body's "rest-and-digest" response, which – as you can probably tell from its nickname – is exactly the opposite of the "fight-or-flight" mode.

- <u>Connectedness</u> – from the spiritual standpoint, breathing is something you have in common with every other person on earth, and focusing your attention on your breath therefore allows you to strengthen your shared interconnection with others (regardless of any physical separation).

Also, take notice that *laughter* shares the exact same four characteristics as deep breathing, because laughter *is* deep breathing. Just be careful to note that genuinely meaningful laughter really only occurs when you're laughing *with* people rather than at them, because our human connections suffer greatly whenever humor comes at someone else's expense.

As for personal expressions of **creativity** (i.e., music, art, writing, dance, etc.), they're potentially even more powerful than physical activity when it comes to stress, due to the freedom they provide. That's because most people really aren't as free as they think they are (even in "free" countries), and let's take a look at why that's true.

Many of us clearly remember that as kids we had the ability to enthusiastically play almost anywhere, any time, and with anyone or anything, because our imaginations were so active. Even sitting in someone's yard or in a park with nothing more than some twigs, leaves, and pebbles, we could amuse ourselves for hours by creating entire worlds full of characters and stories, right from our own minds.

An unfortunate thing happens to most folks as we get older, though. We start to be progressively less free in our personal expressions, as we increasingly worry about what's "realistically" possible, and – even more unfortunately – what *other* people will think of us. We also become so concerned with our daily roles (parent, spouse, employee, manager, etc.) and our personal responsibilities (rent, food, utility bills, and so on), that we lose much of our ability to be spontaneous and playful, which results in the figurative – and sometimes literal – closing of doors.

Maybe even more importantly, though, we also start making a lot of assumptions, many of which aren't even remotely close to being correct. For instance:

- we assume there's no time to play any more, because we assume that play can't simultaneously coexist with things like work, school, errands, etc.

- we come to believe that creativity is one of those things where either you have it or you don't, and that if you don't have it, it can't be developed

- we become overly self-conscious and mistake-avoidant, fearing our "errors" will result in embarrassment and humiliation

- we assume there's only one "right" way of doing things, and that all other options have ceased to exist

- we become afraid of the unknown, rather than excitedly seeking to explore it.

Because of these assumptions, our previously abundant alternatives seem to vanish, leaving us feeling stuck, trapped, and even hopeless. That's why returning to a "childlike" mindset (which is very different from a *childish* mindset) is so valuably important for all of us, and it's also why creative expressions can be so powerful for relieving distress.

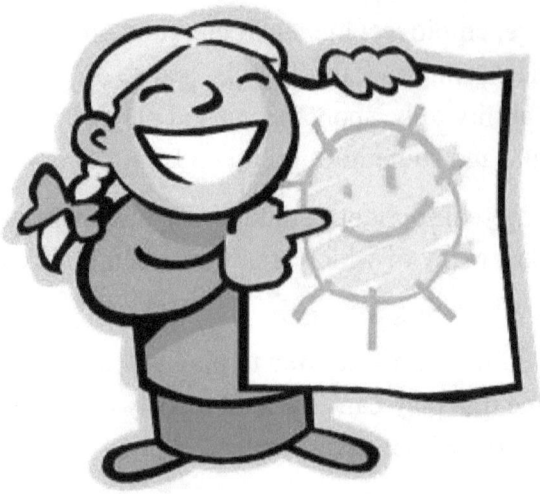

Figure 3.3 – Personal Creativity

Additionally, there are many creative forms of expression which don't even require the use of words, which further helps to release long-held concerns from your conscious *and* subconscious awareness. These methods also dramatically improve your ability to simultaneously combine:

- playfulness

- non-judgmental thought patterns

- the encouragement and development of creativity (which really does exist in everybody)

- the realization of essentially unlimited options (which are much easier to see when you're not forcing yourself into somebody else's expectations of what that you "should" be like).

As a result, doors re-open. Multiple opportunities re-appear. You feel hope<u>ful</u>, instead of hopeless. And all of that because you're freely and openly expressing yourself. In the meantime, you'll also be expanding your personal comfort zones by exploring new territories and developing new talents and skills, and *that's* a wonderful thing.

Along the way, please keep in mind when filling your toolbox to choose stress coping strategies that work for <u>you</u>. Seriously, think about that for a minute. How many times have you heard folks recommending stress coping strategies that they described as being amazingly effective, but which didn't work for you at all?

For me, the first example which immediately comes to mind here is a hot bath, because I've been told my several people that hot baths "melt away" their stress. However, if I take a hot bath when I'm feeling genuinely stressed, I just end up feeling hot and stressed! That's why your stress coping toolbox has to be filled with *your* most effective tools, and if someone else's tools don't work for you, that's totally okay. Just remember that the more your tools work for you, the more relaxed you'll be during all of life's situations, including circumstances which may seem entirely beyond your control (such as natural disasters, unexplained illnesses, etc.).

MOVING FURTHER UPSTREAM

Let's say you've developed a well-stocked toolbox and you're already using a wide variety of coping strategies similar to those listed earlier in this chapter, but you're still not as far upstream in Irving Zola's swiftly flowing river as you'd like to be. In that case, it's time to revisit the 2nd question you were asked in Chapter 1, regarding the current stressors in your life.

Looking through your list of personal stressors again, see if it contains any of the following four themes which are so common today:

- <u>Time</u> – we all know the feeling of not having enough hours in a day to do everything we feel needs to be done, and whether that's *despite* modern technology or *because of* modern technology remains an enthusiastic debate. Either way, it's certainly not in your favor to accumulate a lengthy list of overdue tasks, and we'll look at several ways to address that in a moment.

- Money – the description for this factor is almost a mirror image of the one above, since we also all know the feeling of not having enough money in the bank to buy everything we feel needs to be bought. Conversely, some folks actually feel stressed because their wealth *exceeds* their money management skills, and we'll address both of these situations shortly.

- Conflict – interpersonal conflict (i.e., conflict between you and someone else) is an extremely common stressor in today's world, and we'll look at it in considerable detail.

- Values – once you choose to move upstream by addressing the major issues like time, money, and conflict, your ultimate success will depend on you identifying and addressing your deepest personal values, because they form the foundation of every other stressor you have. We'll review that here, too.

VALUES

Trying to address things like time, money, and conflict without first addressing your core personal values is a clear case of putting the cart before the horse. Unfortunately, I can't even begin to count the number of times I've seen clients and students trying to somehow acquire more time and money, without first looking at why their current allotment of time and money seemed so scarce to them in the first place.

The first time I noticed that discrepancy was back in college, when my roommate and I had a friend come to our apartment one day and ask, "Hey, do you guys have anything to eat? I don't have any food in my place, and I'm starving." As you may already know, that's a fairly common question among college students, so we figured he just hadn't had the chance to go grocery shopping lately, and we replied, "Sure, there's some stuff in the fridge. Help yourself." Our friend then rummaged through the kitchen and sat down to the table with some leftovers and a glass of juice, at which point he said, "Hey, you guys have gotta come over to my place to hang out tonight, because I just bought a new home entertainment system, and it's amazing!"

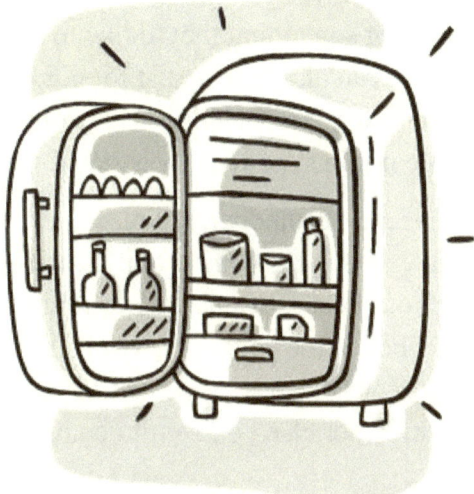

Figure 3.4 – Refrigerator Values

As it turned out, our friend's bare kitchen had nothing to do with him not having enough time to go to the market, but instead was because he'd spent all of his money on home electronics! And while we understood the temptations he felt about some of those "latest and greatest" gadgets, we also knew that our priorities were different than his, because my roommate and I both preferred having an adequate amount of food in the house instead of the latest electronics.

Years later, in my work as a wellness educator, I kept seeing the same type of pattern repeating itself in the lives of my clients and students, whose behavioral choices simply weren't matching their stated priorities. It even got to the point where I started having each person write down a list of his/her most highly esteemed values, and the results were very eye-opening.

When given the task of writing a value list, most people actually begin by writing down many of the same things, including: family, friends, faith, health, freedom, financial stability, meaningful employment, quality education, and so on. I then ask everyone to carry their list around for a few days, so it can be updated whenever they think of something they'd like to add (or change or subtract), and so they can also use the list for guidance whenever faced with major decisions (especially since people often engage in behaviors which are <u>not</u> in sync with their stated values).

From a stress management standpoint, your value/behavior inconsistencies are exceptionally important, because if your actions aren't in line with your deepest values, you *will* cause yourself distress, even if it's below the conscious level. You'll also need to either revise your actions or revise your values in order to bring them all into agreement, or else you won't be able to optimize your well-being.

For a blatant example of how this might play out, let's say you strongly believe that abstaining from alcohol is an essential principle for "living right," and that you do indeed refrain from consuming any alcohol in your own life. At the same time, however, let's also say that you own a liquor store from which you make your living by selling alcohol to other people. Your rationale is that you're just doing what you're good at, and you inherited the business from your parents, and just because you believe in a certain principle doesn't mean you've got to force your views onto other people. However, this is a clear case of your actions not being in sync with your stated values, and even if you don't admit to consciously feeling any distress from that disparity, your body *will* still hold on to it. Plus, you'll also acquire additional distress from having to fend off the claims of hypocrisy coming your way from outside commentators, leaving you in a chronic state of "fight-or-flight" that will exhaust your body's attempts to maintain homeostasis, eventually leading to adverse stress outcomes.

Of course, that's obviously a dramatic example, and it's included here to provide a clear illustration of a value/behavior gap. What's really sneaky, though, is that instead of having one gigantic contradiction like that one, most people instead tend to have several smaller inconsistencies which collectively add up to the exact same stress outcomes.

For my clients, their realization of these discrepancies first becomes apparent to me when they start to revise their value lists. Typically, that means they start adding things they hadn't thought of before, and/or they begin to acknowledge factors they hadn't wanted to previously admit (to themselves and/or to other people), including things like their: reputation, status, lifestyle, luxuries, gratification, personal appearance, privacy, independence, etc.

Fortunately, all of those newly listed values are *self-identified* by each individual person, rather than being bestowed upon them by me or anyone else. And when I ask people how they came to realize their reluctantly-admitted values, their responses are priceless:

- "I've been saying for years that I valued my health, but what I gradually realized is that although I valued *having* my health, I didn't really value *doing* all of the things I needed to do to keep it. That told me I was valuing something else even more than my health, and it looks like

I was more concerned with my lifestyle than my life."

- "The first time I wrote down my list of values, the two things I put at the top were faith and family. In practice, though, I was only spending about one percent of my time on faith and maybe ten percent of my time with my family. That made me take a long look at why my actions didn't seem to match the things that I'd said were so important to me."

- "As a result of this process, I've had to admit to myself that I enjoy *spending* money even more than I enjoy *having* money, and that's why I found myself going deeper and deeper into debt. My previous definition of 'financial security' was just being able to buy whatever I wanted, but I was doing that with credit cards and loans and digging myself a really deep hole. I feel like a sucker for saying this, but I always felt like I deserved what everyone else seemed to have, and I never stopped to think that maybe they're all in just as much debt as I am. I wanted a lot more than I really needed."

- "I kept telling myself that I'd have more free time when I got out of school, or when I got a different job, or when I finished the next project, or whatever. But every time I had that free time, I'd immediately fill it up with something else! Back when I was a little kid, my grandfather told me that the secret to a happy life was hard work, but there's a difference between 'hard' and 'ridiculous,' and if I don't make this transition now, I'm going to be laying next to him in the cemetery a whole lot sooner than I'd planned."

Pretty eye-opening, isn't it? And now that you've listened to these people tell their personal stories, I've got two new questions for you:

- What are *your* core values?

- How do those values affect your stressors?

In all truthfulness, the best chance you have of getting fully upstream is to identify the values underlying your stressors. If you do that, your proactive coping strategies *will* succeed, and you'll be a lot further on your way to resolving your original stressors (rather than merely masking them) than you've ever been before. Plus, adherence to core values also helps to ensure that you're not just replacing your old stressors with new ones (like robbing a bank to pay off debts, for example).

TIME AND MONEY

Perceived shortages of time and money are widely common, to the point that they've already spawned entire books devoted exclusively to managing those two resources better. And although most of those books don't make any attempt to address their readers' values (thereby unfortunately limiting their audience's overall success), they usually do a terrific job of emphasizing other factors which work well for both time and money management. Here are four of those key strategies:

- Keep track of what needs to be done or spent. – It's hard to manage a resource if you don't know how much of it you need, so this is an excellent starting point. Simply write down a list of your time or money commitments (along with any updates whenever necessary), and use that list to help keep track of your resources.

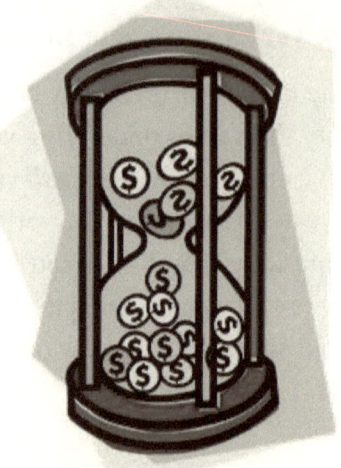

Figure 3.5 – Time and Money

- <u>Prioritize</u>. – Rearrange your commitment list based on your perceived significance of each item, with the most important elements listed at the top (your core values will play a crucial role here). Then, as you begin to manage your list, your personal *style* will affect how you proceed. For instance, some people consider their largest time/money commitments to be their most important ones, and therefore initially focus their energies on completing the most expensive and time-consuming tasks first, followed by addressing the smaller items afterward. Other folks, however, prefer the exact opposite strategy, choosing to take care of the little items in the beginning, so they'll be free to focus on the bigger things later without any distractions. Choose whichever style works best for you.

- <u>Know when to say NO</u>. – Once you've begun to manage a prioritized list of your commitments, it's important to realize that every new intrusion or request has the potential to dramatically affect the commitments you've already made. And since none of us has an unlimited amount of time or money, it's vital to assess the potential impact of any new additions to your list. In other words, since you've already devoted your resources to other obligations, you'll need to evaluate the potential effects of added responsibilities as they arise, so you won't exceed your limits.

- <u>Learn the truth about multi-tasking</u>. – Most of us already know that the more things we try to do "at the same time," the worse we perform on all of them. Quite frankly, that's a collision between quantity and quality that plays itself out every day in these modern times, and yet far too many people unfortunately encourage multitasking as if it's some sort of gift. In truth, although your brain is able *change* its focal point from one thing to another at astonishing speeds, it is *not* capable of focusing on multiple things at the same time. Instead, it first focuses on one thing, and then switches its attention to another thing, and so on. And if you think you're somehow an exception to this principle of human physiology, and that you're the lone person on Earth who's able to multitask, the truth is that you've been deceived! To learn more about the science behind this topic, please feel free to check out either of the following great resources:

    o Christine Rosen, "The Myth of Multitasking," *The New Atlantis*, Number 20, Spring 2008, pp. 105-110.

    o L. Loukopoulos, R. K. Dismukes, & I. Barshi. (2009). The multitasking myth: Handling complexity in real-world operations, Burlington, VT: Ashgate

INTERPERSONAL CONFLICT

The words "conflict" and "stress" have an interesting thing in common, which is that they're both often perceived as being exclusively negative. Interpersonal conflict has even been linked in scientific studies to depression, exhaustion, work disabilities, psychiatric disease, and a host of other adverse health outcomes. In reality, though, *constructive* conflict is a good thing (similar to "eustress" being a positive form of stress), while *destructive* conflict is the one with the adverse outcomes. More on this in a moment.

Along with those two different types of conflict, another determinant of conflict-based health outcomes is the manner in which you handle conflict (i.e., your "conflict style"). Over the years, conflict experts have developed several different ways to classify conflict styles, and there are generally considered to be five main styles:
• <u>dominating/forcing</u> – aggressively competing against foes to determine a clear winner and loser
• <u>obliging/accommodating</u> – self-sacrificing or "giving in" to other people
• <u>avoiding</u> – side-stepping issues completely
• <u>compromising</u> – a "no-win / no-lose" strategy in which opponents meet each other half-way across any differences or divides that exist between them
• <u>integrating/collaborating</u> – problem-solving with others to produce "win-win" outcomes.

Of these five different styles, the one most commonly recommended for resolving conflicts is the collaborative approach, for obvious reasons. After all, if *everyone* "wins," that would certainly sound like a nice way to resolve conflict. In truth, however, the "best" style will likely depend upon each situation's unique environment (e.g., workplace, home, grocery store, etc.), in addition to your core values and past experiences. That's because your conflict style is affected by a multitude of different factors, including cultural influences, personal values, current & past relationships, personal & professional roles, basic temperament, and so on.

For example, my own conflict style was initially influenced by four main factors: the manner in which my parents handled conflict; the area where I grew up (in central New Jersey, about half way between New York City and Philadelphia); the American cultural ideal for males (i.e., strong, rugged, "manly" men); and the sports I played during high school and college (e.g., football and rugby). The combined interplay of these factors resulted in me adopting the winner/loser mindset of the dominating/forcing conflict style, and I'd be lying if I said it worked out well for me.

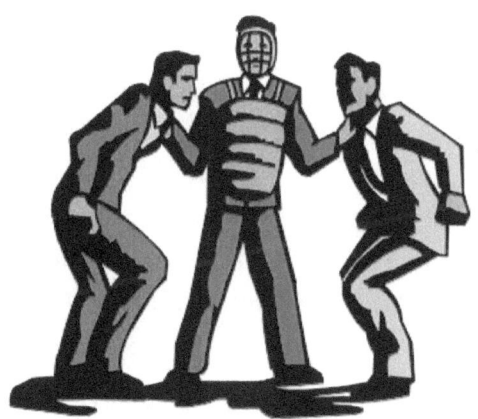

Figure 3.6 – Interpersonal Conflict

In reality, my use of a combative conflict style resulted in enemies, lost friends, "bad blood," and a host of other outcomes which were far less than optimal. My subsequent response, therefore, was mainly to avoid conflicts, but that just resulted in countless missed opportunities. Eventually, I became so frustrated with my inability to maturely handle conflict that I enrolled in a university-based

Conflict Resolution training program, where I finally began to learn the long-overdue life skill of *constructive* conflict management. The timing of that training was also very helpful, by the way, because I started the program at about the same time I became the president of a homeowners' association, and – if there was ever a time in my life when I needed to handle conflict carefully – that was it!

Since then, I've become much better at handling conflict, although I'm still learning as I go. In the meantime, my improved abilities have positioned me a lot further upstream in Irving Zola's swiftly flowing river than I used to be, thereby producing a noticeably positive effect on both my stress outcomes and my interpersonal relationships. I've also become more empathetic and better at communication, because both of those characteristics were addressed by my school's training program, which was one of the best investments I've ever made.

Of course, you might not have any desire to go to school for conflict resolution (or any other field of study), and that's totally okay, especially since many of the things taught in those academic programs are also available via workshops, DVDs, books, and other delivery methods. In fact, my three favorite learning experiences from Conflict Resolution training are widely available elsewhere, and they include:

- Analysis of conflict style: have you ever formally identified your conflict style? Several high-quality questionnaires will allow you to do this for free, and a great example which is available online is the *Adult Personal Conflict Style Inventory.*

- Enhanced communication: *"Difficult conversations: How to discuss what matters most"* is a practical, easy-to-read paperback authored by Stone, Patton, and Heen (most recently updated in 2010 by Penguin Books), and it's an excellent tool for improving communication skills.

- <u>Mediation training</u>: being able to *practice* the role of a neutral, third-party intermediary is tremendously valuable when developing constructive conflict resolution skills, thanks to the hands-on experience you'll gain by working through real-life issues. To find out more about mediation training programs in your area (many of which use creative scheduling to accommodate a wide variety of busy schedules), try contacting the *Association for Conflict Resolution* in Reston, VA (and please note that the subject of this paragraph is "mediation," rather than the "meditation" topic discussed earlier in this chapter).

CHAPTER SUMMARY

Now that you're fully acquainted with proactive and reactive stress management principles, you should feel much more comfortable choosing optimal coping strategies for each stressor you encounter. And to help you strengthen these new habits as you move further upstream in your swiftly flowing river of life, let's use the final chapter to focus on the art and science of behavior change.

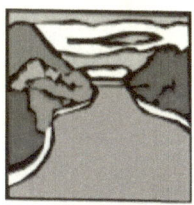

CHAPTER 4
THE REST OF YOUR LIFE STARTS NOW

If you've ever made a New Year's resolution and/or tried to change an old habit, you already know that behavior change can sometimes seem like a formidable task. That idea can also be reinforced by the fancily-named theories used by psychologists to address this topic, including the Transtheoretical Model, Theory of Reasoned Action, Social Cognitive Theory, etc. Fortunately, we're about to simplify five of the most decisive factors affecting behavior change, including: decision making, goal setting, locus of control, self efficacy, and brain control.

DECISION MAKING

Interestingly, two of the most common factors affecting good decision making are on opposite ends of a time-based spectrum: impulsiveness and procrastination.

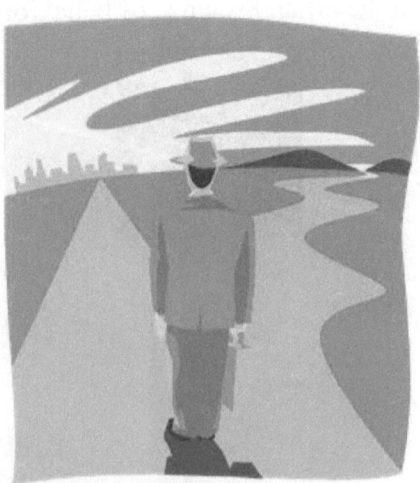

Figure 4.1 – Decision Making

- **Impulsiveness** is particularly challenging when decisions are made *emotionally*, because the emotional parts of the brain will literally overpower the rational parts of the brain, thereby increasing the likelihood of making irrational decisions. To overcome impulsive tendencies, consider using one of the many decision making worksheets, flowcharts, or matrices available online and in bookstores. There are numerous versions available, and the common trait among all of them is that they *slow you down*, which allows your rational brain to reclaim some very valuable turf from your emotional brain. And while the use of a decision making model might feel awkward at first, you'll soon find that once you've used one of those models a few times, the overall process will begin to feel much more comfortable and natural, and you'll soon be making consistently logical decisions.

- **Procrastination** is often linked to a situation known as "analysis paralysis," in which the fear of making a poor decision – and/or the fear of an undesirable outcome – results in apparently making no decision at all (although, as the rock group Rush once famously sang, "If you choose not to decide, you still have made a choice."). To overcome procrastination, be sure to keep in mind the principle of proactive stress management. That is, any time you resolve an original stressor, you're moving further upstream and expanding your comfort margins. So when you address a stressor directly (rather than procrastinating), it becomes a complete non-factor and therefore frees up all of your remaining energy for enjoyment. And life truly feels extraordinary when you're able to "go out and play" without any worries burdening your mind.

GOAL SETTING

A number of formal goal setting methods have been developed over the years, in response to the overly vague goals so often used by far too many people (e.g., "I want to lose weight," "I'd like to be more fit," "I want to decrease my stress," etc.). In each of the preceding examples, for instance, the stated goals are simply too unclear to be helpful, because they don't include enough information – such as timelines and methods – to let you know how or when the goals will be achieved.

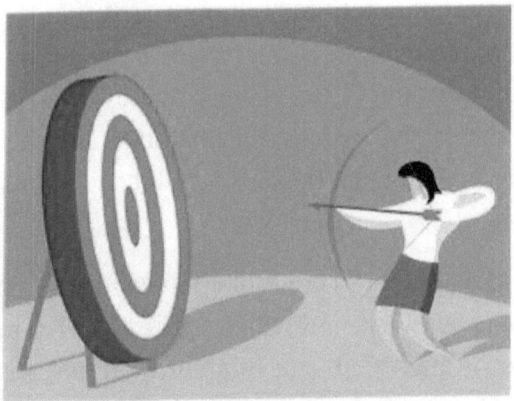

Figure 4.2 – Goal Setting

Conversely, there are several "S.M.A.R.T." goal-setting strategies available, and the version which has been most successfully used by my clients and students is:
• S – Specific
• M – Measurable
• A – Achievable
• R – Relevant
• T – Time-defined

A good example of a SMART goal would be something like, "I'm going to sit and close my eyes for 5 consecutive minutes of quiet meditation, twice per day, 7 days per week, starting tomorrow, and consistently maintaining that for the next 4 weeks." And here's why that's a SMART goal:

- *Specific* activity/method = seated, quiet meditation
- *Measurable* numbers = every day, twice per day, 5 minutes per session
- *Achievable* = "yes; I can do it on my lunch break and before I go to bed"
- *Relevant* = "yes; meditation helps to improve mind control and reduce stress"
- *Time-defined* = starts tomorrow and lasts for 4 weeks.

If you're one of the many people who struggle with setting clearly defined goals, try using the SMART strategy and see what you think. Most folks feel wonderfully relieved when they suddenly start fulfilling their goals, and it's amazing when all of that happens just because they stated their goals a little more clearly.

LOCUS OF CONTROL

Several years ago, when the average price of gasoline jumped up above $4 per gallon, one of the national news agencies sent out reporters to interview people who were filling up their cars at gas stations. One particular consumer got my attention immediately, because he unleashed a televised tirade against Congress, OPEC (Organization of Petroleum Exporting Countries), the President of the United States, and several other international players. What really caught my interest, though, was what he *didn't* say, because he never once mentioned anything that he could have personally done to address his consumption of gasoline. Instead, he focused all of his energies on blaming other people, in a classic case of what psychologists describe as an "external locus of control," which matters a lot more than you might think.

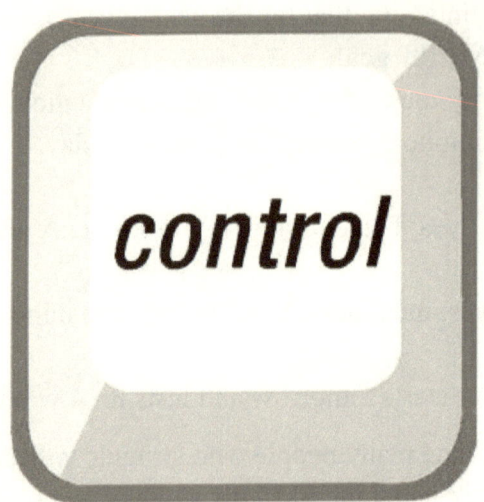

Figure 4.3 – Locus of Control

The word "locus" means "place" (as in "location"), and a person's locus of control is the place where his/her control of life is considered to be centered. In other words, people who have an *external* locus of control have a "victim" mentality, because they believe all of the events in their lives are controlled by outside circumstances (i.e., luck, fate, destiny, etc.). On the other hand, people with an *internal* locus of control have a "contributor" mentality, because they believe the events in their lives are controlled by their own personal behaviors. Overall, most folks actually have a more balanced status which is partially internal and partially external, and – either way – your locus of control is genuinely important because:

- if your position is overly external, you won't try to make any changes in your life because you don't think your efforts will matter

- if your position is overly internal, you'll eventually feel overwhelmed by life, because you feel responsible for *everything*.

The vast majority of my clients and students have a locus of control that's about 2/3 internal and 1/3 external, which means that while they view their personal choices and behaviors as making a big difference in life, they also know that some things (like earthquakes, for instance) are totally beyond their control. That's a great viewpoint to have when trying to change personal behaviors, because it reinforces the fact that you do indeed have the power to greatly influence the direction and outcome of your life, regardless of whatever else is happening in the world.

To learn more about *your* personal locus of control, check out some of the free assessments available online, a great example of which is the *Locus of Control & Attributional Style Test*. There's also a lot of help available for anyone whose locus of control is excessively external or internal, because good counselors and therapists are effectively able to guide their clients into better-balanced approaches in which everyone realizes their personal strengths and limitations. This also brings us back full circle to the topic of perception again, which is an excellent way to introduce the final concepts of self-efficacy and brain control.

SELF-EFFICACY & BRAIN CONTROL

Self-efficacy is a fancy name for something many of us first learned about via a childhood story called, "The Little Engine That Could," in which a little train pulled a heavy load up a mountainside while repeating, "I think I can...I think I can...I think I can." There's also an adult version of this concept that's attributed to the legendary automaker Henry Ford, who was quoted as saying something along the lines of, "Whether you think you can, or you think you can't -- you're right."

Simply put, people with a high degree of self-efficacy have a positive belief in their own capabilities, which means they have a strong faith that they'll be able to accomplish whatever they set out to do. That mindset is also commonly associated with positive "self-talk," since all of us talk to ourselves (out loud or otherwise) continuously. That's why self-efficacy is such a big deal, because when our thoughts are filled with positive messages we inspire ourselves to achieve greater things. On the other hand, if we bombard ourselves with negative messages we limit ourselves to lesser things.

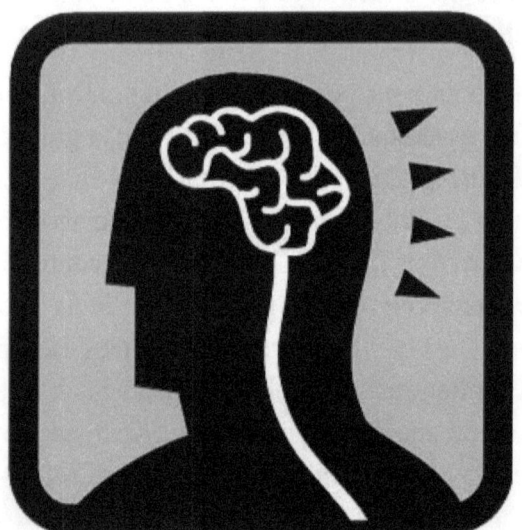

Figure 4.4 – Self-Efficacy & Brain Control

Two fantastic self-efficacy role models in recent years have included the late Randy Pausch (a former professor who skyrocketed to fame with his "Last Lecture") and the late Charlie Wedemeyer (who continued to coach high school football after being diagnosed with – and being dramatically affected by – amyotrophic lateral sclerosis (ALS), also known as Lou Gehrig's disease). These inspirational people were exactly that: inspirational *people*. And they overcame extraordinary adversity in life because they (and their loved ones) kept telling themselves, "I think I can...I think I can...I think I can."

They were right, of course, and the power of their positive faith is just as relevant to you today as it was to them. In fact, even if you're thinking that your habits or behaviors are too firmly entrenched to be changed, the science of neuroplasticity (i.e., the ability of the brain to rewire itself in response to change) *guarantees* that you can transform into everything you've ever wanted to be. And if you have any doubts about that, you owe it to yourself to check out some of the great brain books by Dr. Jeffrey Schwartz from UCLA, including: You Are Not Your Brain; Brain Lock; and The Mind and The Brain.

You'll soon see that *every* change you make is further etched into your neural circuitry each time it's repeated, thereby reinforcing your new habits and behaviors while simultaneously overwriting the old ones. That means you can successfully cope with any stressor, firmly position yourself far upstream, and happily avoid ever having to wake up with your mouth locked shut from stress.

That's the life you're fully capable of having, and the one you can proactively achieve.

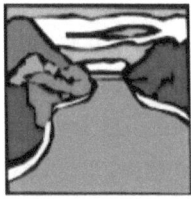

ACKNOWLEDGEMENTS

I'm sincerely grateful to all of the following people, whose positive impact on this book has been invaluable:
• the outstanding professionals who reviewed my early manuscripts, including: Wieland D. Chong, Jr., JD; Nicole A. Kerr, MPH, RD; and David Klinger, PhD
• the innumerable students, clients, coworkers, and professors with whom I've worked over the years
• my wonderful wife
• my wise parents.

I'd also like to pay special tribute to:
• Dr. Glenn Richardson, who wisely introduces all of his students to the work of Irving Zola, and who understands better than anyone that sometimes just walking across the street can change your life forever. Many thanks for sharing Irving's story and your own.
• Dr. Joaquin Fenollar, who does a better job of living with passionate integrity than anyone else I've ever met.

Aloha

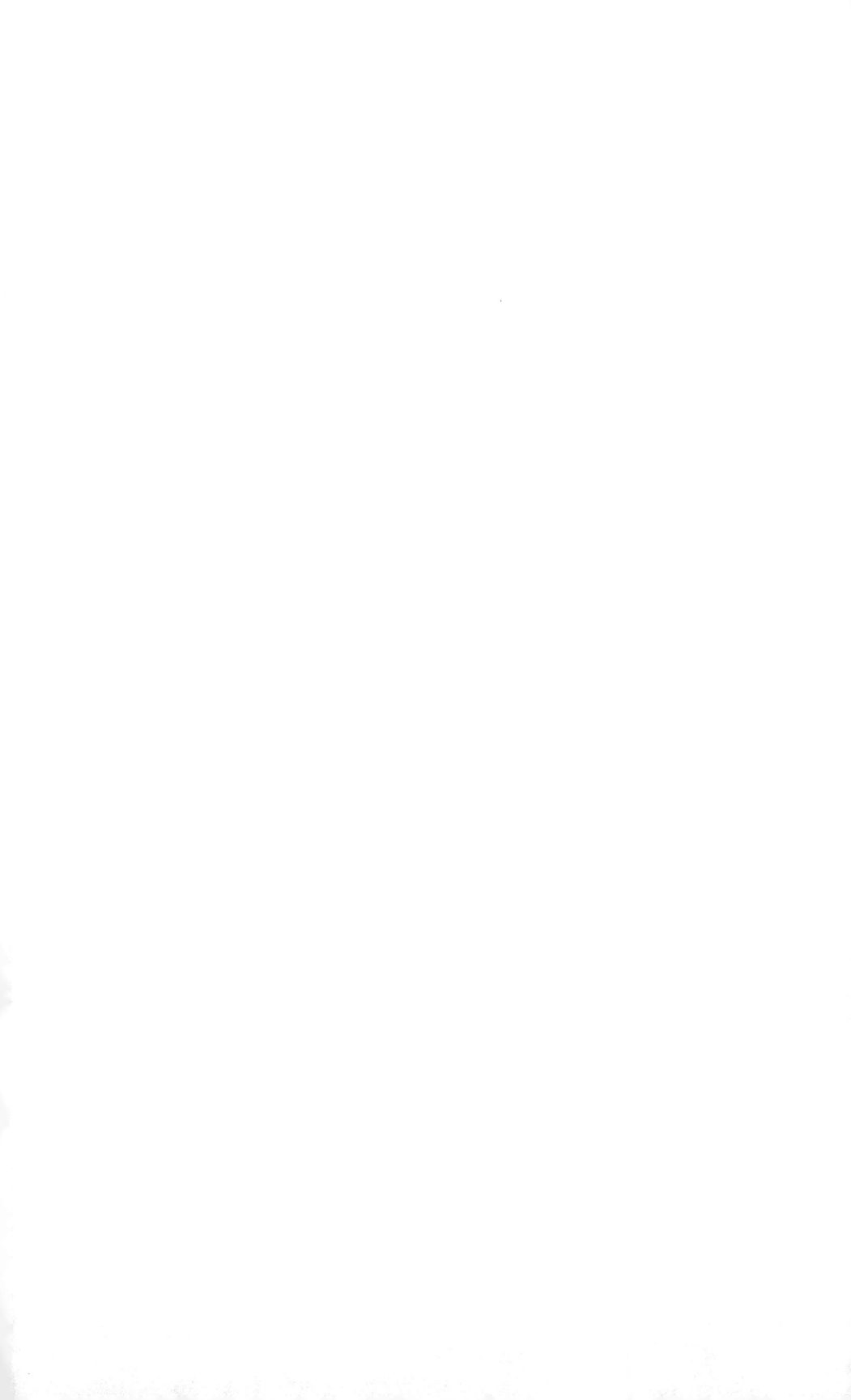

www.ingramcontent.com/pod-product-compliance
Lightning Source LLC
Chambersburg PA
CBHW030537290526
45786CB00004B/1747